A Guide Through The Gluten-Free World

DR. HOWARD PEIPER

TABLE OF CONTENTS

INTRODUCTION

If we love to eat wheat but hate the way it makes us feel, odds are we are among the 30 percent of the population who are intolerant to a protein molecule called gluten. Gluten is found primarily in grains, including wheat (spelt, durum and semolina are types of wheat), barley and rye. Oats are grains and do not have gluten. However, oats often become cross-contaminated when they are planted in fields that have grown wheat. The popular solution for gluten intolerance is to follow a gluten-free lifestyle, eliminating the offending protein to reduce adverse reactions.

The real challenge with gluten intolerances is cross contamination. Gluten is hidden in countless consumer products, from chewing gum to medications and cosmetics to the glue on postage stamps. This book will help familiarize us with hidden sources of gluten and various healthy, gluten-free recipes.

THE BIG PICTURE

The food we eat is the single most important factor impacting our health. Unfortunately, for many of us, our health is not good. We do not make the right choices. Today, two out of three American adults are overweight, and of those, 36 percent are obese. Most of us eat too much refined wheat and sugar. Fewer than 24 percent of us eat enough fruits and vegetables. Sadly, we pass these habits on to our children. One in six kids is overweight, and obesity is the leading health threat. More than 90 million people in the United States live with at least one chronic disease.

We need to take responsibility for our own health. Being in good health improves our quality of life, because good health provides the energy to do the things we enjoy. Too many people believe it is easier to take medication than to engage in healthy eating and exercise. This medical community reinforces this unhealthy belief. Their goal in caring for patients with chronic conditions is all too often to find treatments (in the form of medicine) that produce fewer side effects. In contrast, what their patients really need is prevention-focused healthcare. The significant role of diet in the development and treatment of chronic disease is undervalued in this country. Our food choices have upset the body's balance. We are anxious, overstimulated and inflamed. The inflammation weakens the immune system. A weak immune system is the trigger for chronic disease. Strengthening our immune system is the key to health and vitality.

A healthy person has an internal chemistry that is in balance, so his or her immune system is strong. A healthy immune system protects us from chronic inflammation, which causes not only arthritis and body aches, but also digestive disorders, allergies, asthma, thyroid problems and other chronic diseases, such as Alzheimer's disease, cancer, diabetes and heart disease. We need to eat smart to neutralize the inflammation in our body that causes disease.

FOOD SENSITIVITY

Food sensitivity is the general term used to refer to individualistic adverse reactions to food or food components (usually proteins). Reactions that involve the immune system are called food allergies, and those that may or may not involve the immune system are called food intolerances.

Food Allergies

A food allergy is an immediate hypersensitive immunologic response to a food protein and involves the immediate formation of allergen-specific immunoglobulin E (IgE) antibodies, with symptoms occurring shortly after eating the offending food. For example, a peanut allergy is an immediate immunologic response to the peanut protein. True food allergies equal to only a fraction of all food sensitivities. Approximately 90 percent of all IgE-mediated food allergies are caused by: peanuts, tree nuts, milk, eggs, soybeans, fish, shellfish and wheat.

Food Intolerances

Food intolerance is a delayed hypersensitivity and can be caused by the absence of specific chemicals or enzymes needed to digest a food substance. It can also be caused by the body's responses to certain food components, both natural and artificial. For example, lactose intolerance is caused by the body's inability to produce enough lactase (enzyme) to break down the lactose present in milk.

The Gluten Sensitivity Spectrum

Gluten, a protein molecule with a unique sequence and structure, is found in wheat, barley and rye, but not in oats, corn or rice. Gluten sensitivity enteropathy (any disease of the intestine) is associated with a variety of symptoms and health conditions. Gluten sensitivity includes wheat and gluten allergies, wheat intolerance and gluten intolerance. There are two types of gluten intolerance: nonceliac and celiac disease.

Celiac Disease

Celiac disease is a genetic autoimmune disease that results from the inability to tolerate gluten. When people with celiac disease consume gluten, their body launches an immune attack on the lining of the small intestine. The small intestine is lined with tiny, finger-like projections called villi, which secrete digestive enzymes and absorb nutrients. Celiac disease can damage or destroy the villi, resulting in the poor absorption of nutrients.

Celiac disease is the most prevalent chronic autoimmune disease, and because it is genetic, it runs in families. It can manifest itself anytime during a person's life and often becomes active for the first time after experiencing stress, pregnancy, surgery or a viral infection.

More than 210 symptoms are associated with celiac disease, and almost every single person has a different set of symptoms. The most common symptoms include: diarrhea, gas, bloating, vomiting, constipation, nausea, skin irritation, anemia, weight loss, chronic fatigue, weakness, joint pain, muscle cramps, neurologic complaints, migraine headaches, body aches, thyroid problems and concentration and memory problems. Malabsorption caused by celiac disease can cause serious side effects on many other organs of the body and can lead to other autoimmune diseases: cancer, diabetes and heart disease.

The only accepted treatment for celiac disease is a gluten-free lifestyle, which is a life free of wheat, rye and barley. Gluten is one of the most common ingredients in processed foods and is found in everything from soup stock to soy sauce to butterscotch morsels. Therefore, it is important that people with celiac disease read food ingredient labels and be extremely careful when eating food prepared outside the home.

NonCeliac Gluten Intolerance

Some people who experience distress when eating products containing gluten, and those who show improvement after following a gluten-free lifestyle, may have nonceliac gluten intolerance instead of celiac disease. Nonceliac gluten intolerance generally worsens over time, but, unlike celiac disease, there may be no damage to the small intestine. Gluten intolerance is caused by a defect in the body's ability to digest the gliadin protein in gluten; humans do not have the proper enzymatic capacity to completely break down the gliadin protein into small, digestible molecules. Inflammation occurs and damage to the intestinal wall can cause leaky gut syndrome.

Nonceliac gluten intolerance is also a delayed hypersensitivity. Symptoms of this type of food sensitivity include gas, intermittent diarrhea, constipation, irritable bowel syndrome (IBS), skin rashes, migraine headaches, arthritis, thyroid problems, neurologic problems, asthma, allergies, sinus infections and an unproductive cough. As with celiac disease, there are more than 210 symptoms associated with nonceliac gluten intolerance and almost everyone has a different set of symptoms.

Wheat or Gluten Allergy

True wheat or gluten allergy symptoms can range from mild discomfort to the potentially life-threatening, and symptoms typically occur within minutes to an hour after eating the offending foods. Common symptoms of a wheat or gluten allergy include: skin irritations, such as rashes, hives and eczema and gastrointestinal symptoms, such as nausea, diarrhea and vomiting.

It is important to understand the difference between celiac disease, gluten intolerance and wheat allergy. Celiac disease is not a food allergy; it is an autoimmune disease. Food allergies, including wheat allergy, are conditions that people can grow out of and that do not destroy the body's tissues. This is not the case with celiac disease. Celiac disease is an autoimmune condition that puts the patient at risk for other autoimmune conditions, such as thyroid disease, type 1 diabetes, joint diseases (RA) and liver diseases (Hepatitis). Because wheat allergy and nonceliac gluten intolerance are not autoimmune conditions, people who have food allergies and intolerances may not be at increased risk to develop an autoimmune condition, but they may still suffer physical consequences because of the immune system's inflammatory reaction to gluten.

THE MANY MASKS OF GLUTEN SENSITIVITY

Gluten sensitivity is a chameleon-like disease. Instead of confining itself to one area of the body, it can develop in many areas and in many different, unsuspected ways.

The condition's ability to hide behind a variety of symptoms makes it difficult, but not impossible, to diagnose correctly. Without the correct diagnosis, it is impossible for a doctor to prescribe the correct remedy, which in the case of gluten sensitivity is one thing: a gluten-free lifestyle. Prescribing the incorrect remedy can often cause even more complicated problems than the original disease!

Misdiagnosis, because of gluten sensitivity's ability to masquerade and piggyback onto the symptoms of other diseases and disorders, can cause devastating effects. Not only are misdiagnosed relegated to "living with" a disease, but living with this condition can lead to severe consequences: the irreversible crippling of rheumatoid arthritis (RA), bone loss and breakage, infection, dementia or even death.

Gluten sensitivity has been associated with several non-celiac, autoimmune conditions, such as: autoimmune hepatitis, immune thyroid disorders, dermatitis herpetiformis (a severe skin condition), autoimmune cardiomyopathy (a form of heart disease), lymphoma (cancer of the blood), insulin-dependent diabetes, Lupus and RA.

Neurological disorders typically lead to diverse problems, such as: lack of muscle coordination, unexplained and severe headaches and psychiatric problems that are exemplified by bizarre behavior. Not all neurological disorders can be attributed to a gluten sensitivity, of course. But gluten sensitivity can cause the same symptoms. When symptoms persist and medical remedies are ineffective, it may be time to consider gluten intolerance.

ALCOHOLISM – GLUTEN INTOLERANCE

Many alcoholics have hidden food sensitivities particularly to foods from which alcohol has been derived; these include wheat, corn, yeast, grapes, sugar, fructose and potato. It is estimated that 80% of alcoholics are gluten intolerant. Alcoholics improve greatly when all grains and gluten products are removed from their diets.

Alcoholics also suffer from hypoglycemia, low blood sugar and blood sugar instability. Individuals tend to experience cravings when they are hypoglycemic and as a result experience sugar, carbohydrate and alcohol cravings, mood swings, irritability, gluten intolerance, brain fog and adrenal exhaustion. These conditions can be remedied by eating a nutrient-dense diet that contains plenty of protein, healing fats and fiber from organically grown leafy green vegetables.

The commonly held view of alcoholics as psychologically sick or simple lazy and irresponsible is simply not correct. For some time, it has been known that many alcoholics suffer from hypoglycemia or low blood sugar levels. He or she drinks to relieve standard hypoglycemic symptoms of depression, tension, irritability, tiredness, inability to think, and so on. The alcohol gives a blood sugar boost which acts as positive reinforcement, conveying relaxation, increased energy and in general, a reversal of the unpleasant hypoglycemic sensations. Over a period, the typical alcoholic displaces what little nutritious food he or she may still consume in favor of alcohol, until the diet is even lower in protein and nutrients, further setting the stage for more hypoglycemia and, therefore, alcoholism.

The same progression can occur for a person who takes his or her first drinks due to true psychological problems. Long after the original psychological cause is gone, the physiological alcoholic addiction remains. Malnutrition usually precedes alcoholism and is aggravated by it.

The real worry about modern alcoholism treatment is its woeful long-term success rate. That means we need to be vigilant with every aspect of mental, emotional and physical well-being. If we want long-term sobriety, we need to look at our diet and take supplements to help curb sugar cravings and boost our Dopamine neurotransmitter, the center for satisfaction and reward.

We can recover from alcoholism, but we cannot recover from hypoglycemia overnight, in a few short weeks we can feel much better. We can banish symptoms and correct the underlying metabolic errors by following a healthy diet and taking some nutritional supplements. We will need to give up foods containing refined sugar. That means virtually all sweets, biscuits, ice cream, etc. We may not want them when we've been drinking, but most alcoholics begin to crave sweets as soon as we go on the wagon. We sometimes pendulum between AA meetings and Overeaters Anonymous meetings.

Have we ever wondered about the similarities between alcohol and sugar? Both are carbohydrates with no nutritional value, all we get from them is calories. Both are absorbed directly into the bloodstream, and both can cause memory blackouts and intense cravings. In addition to sugars, the recommended recovery from alcoholism diet temporarily eliminates dairy products and wheat. Both are highly allergenic and one or frequently contribute to problems of alcohol allergy/addiction.

The best diet for the alcoholic is one that eliminates ALL GLUTEN, wheat and processed grains, soy, soda, sugar, potato, and processed carbohydrates. A nutrient-dense diet high in B vitamins, rich in clean protein, plenty of leafy greens and vegetables, low-sugar fruit and healthy, healing fats is the best diet for a recovering alcoholic.

Protein and fat help prevent blood sugar fluctuations, increase energy, fuel the brain and eliminate cravings. Protein, rich in amino acids provides fuel and helps balance brain chemistry by boosting the levels of mood regulating neurotransmitters. The first 40 grams of protein eaten every day goes to rebuilding the immune system. If we are not rebuilding our immune system, we will have a hard time rebuilding our brain chemistry to be happy and think straight. We need to change our thinking to change our feelings (emotions) to change our behavior towards drinking alcohol.

BRAIN HEALTH AND GLUTEN INTOLERANCE

The causes of depression, anxiety, migraines, or loss of balance are frequently unidentified or unknown. This is often the case for several neurological and psychological disorders. Ongoing research points out that many cases of neurological disorders (depression, anxiety, balance problems, etc.) may reflect adverse impact of gluten on the brain for those who have undiagnosed gluten intolerance and celiac disease.

The well-known or classic symptoms of celiac disease such as weight loss, diarrhea, malabsorption, anemia and abdominal bloating are no longer the norm for diagnosis of celiac disease and gluten intolerance. Current research shows that symptoms frequently present with minimal or no gastrointestinal symptoms, but instead affects other organs like the brain and skin.

Neurological and psychological disorders linked with gluten sensitivity and celiac disease are numerous. These include seizure disorders, neuropathy/ nerve pain, tingling and numbness, schizophrenia, depression, migraine, anxiety, ADD/ ADHD, autism, multiple sclerosis, myasthenia gravis, myopathy or muscle weakness, white matter lesions, and ataxia/ balance problems and cerebellar degeneration. The cerebellum is the back part of the brain that is directly involved with balance, movement and body awareness. Dementia has also been linked with gluten intolerance.

Diagnosis of celiac disease has historically focused on small intestine biopsies that show destruction of the villi (microscopic fingerlike projections) in the small intestine that absorb nutrients. Healthy normal tissue appears like a thick heavy shag carpet, but in untreated celiac disease, the villi are flattened like a worn-out thin Berber carpet. This leads to the classic diarrhea, weight loss, malabsorption, and anemia problems seen in celiac disease.

This active inflammatory process from gluten in the gut may trigger some profound changes in the brain and immune system causing symptoms outside of the gut. The **brain** indeed suffers stress due to the complex relationship of the brain-gut axis, causing mental and emotional dysfunction.

Gliadin, a compound found in gluten, causes increased **intestinal permeability** in all individuals, healthy or not. Gluten intolerance researchers identified that all individuals experienced an upregulation of zonulin followed by opening of the doors or "tight junctions" between cells, i.e. it caused **leaky gut syndrome**. Zonulin is a protein that modulates the how permeable the tight junctions are between the digestive tracts cell walls.

The breach in the intestinal barrier known as leaky gut syndrome is hypothesized to affect the **blood-brain barrier**. Research suggests that this breach in the gut lining compromises the protective barrier around the brain which allows gluten proteins or peptides to cross into the brain creating an upset neuro-immune system. This leads to neurological inflammation causing psychological and neurological symptoms.

Remember that the typical GI symptoms are no longer considered the norm for gluten intolerance. Instead, neurological symptoms like depression, anxiety, poor focus, brain fog, seizures, loss of balance, ADD/ADHD, forgetfulness, numbness, and tingling occurs. In fact, the Lancet medical journal in 1998 described periodic trouble with loss of balance as the most common symptom of gluten intolerance regardless of intestinal symptoms. Thus, if a health care provider is not aware of this presentation or not thinking about it, gluten sensitivity may easily be missed, unrecognized, and untreated or labeled as an idiopathic cause. Research shows that as many as 57 percent of those with neurological disorders from unknown causes test positive for gluten intolerance.

A GLUTEN-FREE LIFESTYLE, THE HEALTHY LIFESTYLE

People underappreciate the many health benefits gained by converting to a gluten-free lifestyle, if done properly. All we have to do is examine our society to see the effects of poor dietary habits. Highly processed foods, high caloric intake, foods with high fat content and quick-fix carbohydrates all contributed to a meteoric rise in obesity rates. While the intent of a gluten-free lifestyle is to prevent gluten-induced health disorders, other benefits for our health will result as well.

WHAT NOT TO EAT

Gluten, as we now know, is a protein found in wheat, rye and barley. It is also in less commonly known cereals, such as: spelt, kamut, couscous, bulgar, farina matzo, seitan, semolina and graham flour. These are the cereals that must be avoided in order to maintain a gluten-free lifestyle.

Many other processed food products can contain gluten as a result of added wheat starch or other, hidden ingredients. For example, soy sauce and processed meats are two examples that contain gluten within their ingredient lists. It is important to become knowledgeable about what foods often do and do not have gluten and which ones don't.

Accidental gluten ingestion is common because of hidden gluten in many foods. Creamed vegetables typically contain gluten, as do malted foods. Thickeners, sauces and marinades are other common foods that contain gluten. Anything that contains wheat starch (a common additive) contains gluten. It is very important to check labels and ask dining establishments about our food options if we are at all unsure about the content.

Gluten Foods

Breading • Broth • Malt, typically from barley or corn • Coating Mixes • Communion Wafers • Crab Cakes • Croutons • Hydrolyzed Vegetable Protein (wheat) • Imitation Bacon • Imitation Seafood • Meat Substitutes (Tofurky) • MSG • Rice Dream (processed with barley) • Pastas • Roux • Sausages (some) • Self-basting Poultry • Soy-based Veggie Burgers • Soy Sauce • Stuffing • Tamari • Textured Vegetable Protein • Vital Wheat Gluten (found in imitation meats) • Ricola Cough Drops • Emergen-C (raspberry and mixed berry flavor only) • Brown Rice Syrup • Bran • Dry Roasted Nuts (processing agents may contain wheat) • Crackers • Pretzels • Ice Cream Cones • Ice Cream (if it contains gluten as a binder or in added ingredients, such as cookie dough) • Barbecue Sauce • Pie Shells • Oat-derived Ingredients (in cosmetics or shampoos)

WHAT TO EAT

Bread and pasta products that are considered gluten-free most commonly include those made with rice, corn, potato and soy. Other, less common grains that are safe to ingest include: amaranth, quinoa, sorghum, millet and buckwheat. Other gluten-free products include: an array of seeds, nuts and beans, tapioca and nut flours.

Gluten-Free Not Always the Answer

A gluten-free lifestyle is the easy solution to one problem – gluten sensitivity. But the human body is a complex mechanism, a sum of our environment, the food we eat and genetics. Often, all these conditions predispose us to concurrent problems that are similar in nature. This is especially true about autoimmune diseases. If we have an immune reaction to one type of food, we may experience cross-reactivity to other foods.

Cross-reactivity is a condition in which the autoimmune antibodies our body generates mistakes other food protein for the ones we cannot tolerate. When we experience a cross-reaction to other foods, the effect on our body is the same as if we ingested gluten.

If going on a gluten-free lifestyle fails to bring the results we anticipate, we need to eliminate the following foods (one at a time, in the order given), because we may be experiencing cross-reactivity.

Dairy - Eliminate all dairy products from cows.

Nightshades - Tomatoes, white potatoes, eggplant, peppers and tobacco are a class of plants that have a protein called lectin, which is similar to gluten.

Peanuts - Legumes also have a high content of lectin.

Carrageenan – A food additive and thickening agent.

Corn and Soy - While corn and soy products are generally used as a substitute grain for those with celiac and gluten sensitivity. Remember more than 50 percent of all corn and 90 percent of all soy is genetically modified.

WHAT TO DRINK –
ALKALINE WATER

One common factor with gluten allergy and intolerance is an overly acidic GI tract. This acid overload occurs from the intestines all the way to the esophagus. This acidic state can cause damage to the intestines, resulting in nutritional deficiencies.

Celiac disease diagnosis is usually based on symptoms of fatigue, low energy, digestive problems, muscle cramps, leg tingling, skin rash, iron deficiency, mouth ulcers, and even seizures.

These symptoms often lead to secondary issues including osteoporosis, cancer of the intestines, miscarriages, and autoimmune diseases. Some children experience delayed lack of growth and development due to deficient nutritional absorption.

A gluten free diet is essential. An alkaline diet is equally important. Why? Because alkaline foods protect the intestines from acid overload.

In addition to eating alkaline foods, research shows that drinking freshly-made, ionized Alkaline Water is vital for optimal intestinal protection.

When both alkaline food and ionized Alkaline Water are consumed in abundance, the GI tract can carry normal bacteria again, which aid in digestion. A supplement of probiotics along with ionized Alkaline Water can support the healing process and continued nutritional wellness.

What is Alkaline Water?

Our body is about 70% water, and is like a swimming pool. If the water in our body is not maintained at a proper alkaline pH level, it becomes acidic and starts to break down.

Acidosis and toxemia in our body are the root causes of most diseases and health problems. Drinking Alkaline Water helps neutralize body acid in our cells, fluids, tissues and organs leading to increased oxygen levels and energy!

A healthy body functions best when it is slightly alkaline. One of the easiest ways to achieve this ideal state is by drinking adequate amounts of Alkaline Water with an 8.0 to 10.0 pH level.

However, BEWARE of Alkaline Water in plastic bottles! Why? Simply put, we would be shocked to know that when water is placed in plastic bottles, it tends to leach out toxic resins and chemical compounds from the plastic. Also, the alkaline strength of the water (a beneficial part) will significantly weaken in the weeks and months it takes to get delivered to stores.

For example, at the bottling plant, Alkaline Water in plastic bottles may start out at a healthy 9.5 pH level. However, harsh environmental factors such as exposure to light, extreme temperature changes and long travel times cause the "alkaline" water to weaken to a lower pH level of 8.0, 7.0 or even a pH level that is slightly acidic!

Therefore, the best way for most of us to get ultra-pure, healthy Alkaline Water is to install a top-quality water ionizer in our kitchen that can produce higher pH levels. This enables families to drink as much safe, freshly-made ionized Alkaline Water as they want or need.

Make Sure We Drink Water With All 3 A's

To fully combat gluten allergy and intolerance along with Celiac disease, the water we drink must be or have all 3 A's:

- **<u>A</u>live** with Oxygen, Minerals & Molecular Hydrogen

- **<u>A</u>lkaline** with pH adjustments from 7.5 to 10.0 or slightly higher

- **<u>A</u>ntioxidant** with millions of antioxidants in every glass

Below are just some of the many benefits that <u>A</u>live, <u>A</u>lkaline Water with maximum <u>A</u>ntioxidant properties can help our body to achieve and enjoy.

> ➤ Counteract free radicals

> - Delay or stop cell damage
> - Cleanse organs including colon
> - Lubricate muscles & joints
> - Slow down the aging process
> - Boost our immune system
> - Lower risk of many serious diseases

Clearly, every family (and even their pets) should be drinking this very special, ionized **WATER FOR WELLNESS**.

(Please see Helpful Resource Directory for the Ionizer company I recommend)

CROSS CONTAMINATION

When we are brand-new to the gluten-free lifestyle, it is difficult to imagine two things: one, how little gluten it actually takes to make us sick; and two, where that gluten can hide. Gluten cross-contamination —contamination of our gluten-free food with gluten in quantities enough to make us ill — can occur in a variety of different places, including our own kitchen. It also can occur in packaged foods, even those that say "gluten-free" on the packaging.

How can we guard against cross-contamination? Well, we need to know how and where it occurs. Once we have a handle on that, we can prevent it successfully, in most cases anyway.

Some people react more frequently than others to gluten cross-contamination. Even if we are more sensitive, we can still protect ourselves. Here is a list of the most common places gluten cross-contamination occurs:

Left-over gluten in a newly gluten-free kitchen. A gluten-free lifestyle has a huge learning curve, and when you are a complete neophyte, it is tough to know exactly what to do to de-gluten the kitchen completely. Left-over gluten is one of the main reasons people who begin the diet report that they feel great for a few days, but then feel awful for a day or two, even though they are eating gluten-free. Most likely, they have been glutened (experienced recurring symptoms from foods they mistakenly thought were gluten-free) by left-over gluten in their own kitchens.

It can be tough to share a kitchen between gluten and gluten-free foods. It takes full dedication and lots of diligence from every member of the household, not just from the gluten-free member/members. If we do not have that dedication and buy-in from everyone, those who need to be gluten-free almost certainly will continue to suffer from symptoms.

Restaurant meals, even meals billed as "gluten-free". Many restaurants do a decent job of producing gluten-free meals for their customers with celiac disease and gluten sensitivity. But in the vast majority of cases, they are preparing our gluten-free food in the main kitchen, and it can be difficult to prevent cross-contamination in that environment. We can help by making certain the chef understands exactly what we need to make our meal safe. But any time we eat out, we are taking a risk.

Food from a friend or relative's kitchen that is not quite gluten-free enough. It takes most people several months — at least — to get a handle on all they need to do to stay gluten-free. It is highly recommended we never eat food prepared by a friend or a relative unless we are standing there, watching them make it. (And even then, be cautious!) Otherwise, we run the risk of them using contaminated kitchen utensils or cookware to make the food, or even worse, adding an unsafe ingredient unknowingly. It may be rough to tell our friends and relations we will not eat their food, but it is certainly rougher to experience full-blown gluten symptoms just because we did not want to hurt their feelings.

'Gluten-Free'-labeled products. Most people assume that something labeled "gluten-free" is completely free of gluten, but that is not true. Most foods carrying a gluten-free label still contain a tiny amount of gluten, and some people react even to that tiny amount. In addition, the more of these foods we eat, the more gluten we consume and the greater our chance of having a reaction.

Guarding against gluten cross-contamination can seem like it is going to be a full-time job. It is one we need to couple with learning exactly what foods are gluten-free and what foods contain gluten. But believe it or not, there will come a time when it is second nature to us, and our health improves so much that it is unquestionably worth it.

THINK ABOUT FIDO

While most domestic pets are not strictly "celiac" (only Irish Setters have been shown to suffer from this condition), many pets are grain-sensitive on some level. Most of the time, us owners attribute their health problems to other causes, when all that we need is to simply change the daily menu.

Gluten and How It Affects Our Pets

Gluten is a generic term used to describe the proteins found in wheat and other cereal grains. It constitutes a mixture of proteins classified into two groups, called prolamines and glutelins.

In true grain intolerances, an immune response occurs when gluten is consumed and the villi, tiny hair-like projections in the small intestine that absorb nutrients from food, are damaged. Damaged villi do not effectively absorb basic nutrients: proteins, carbohydrates, fats, vitamins, minerals and, in some cases, water and bile salts.

Wheat, barley, rye and oats are excluded when following a "gluten-free diet." Most evidence implicates wheat as the most problematic food. One school of thought is that genetically modified (GM) grains are especially risky for the gluten intolerant. Studies show that when butterflies and other species come in contact with pollen from genetically modified crops, they suffer a number of health problems and genetic mutations eventually occur. It is possible that a similar thing happens when other species consume GM grains — especially species whose systems are not designed to cope with a grain overload in the first place.

Signs of Gluten Intolerance in Pets

Consumption of glutenous grains in sensitive pets can lead to:

Chronic GI upset – Intermittent or continuing diarrhea and/or constipation, including mucusy stools. Vomiting may also occur in more severe cases.

Dermatitis – Chronic dry and flaky skin, hair loss, redness, bumps, rashes and constant scratching are classic signs of a food intolerance.

Chronic ear infections – Over-consumption of grain can lead to a buildup of excess sugars in the system. This, in turn, can contribute to yeast overgrowth that leads to dark, smelly waxy debris in the ears, head shaking and scratching.

Other health problems that may be related to food intolerances, such as grain sensitivity, include: arthritis, epilepsy, abnormal behavior, allergic and inflammatory reactions (including inhalant allergies due to a compromised immune system), pancreatitis, hepatitis (as well as an increased susceptibility to infection), Cushing's, Addison's and thyroid problems. Of course, not all of these conditions are directly related to grain consumption. However, the overload of grain in most modern commercial pet diets is thought to deplete animals' natural state of good health over time, leaving them more susceptible to these problems.

Know If Your Pets Are Grain-Intolerant

When several of the above signs are present, a couple of options exist to definitively determine if grain-sensitivity is the culprit.

Diagnostic blood tests are available, but they are not always completely accurate – and can be very costly.

An elimination diet is one of the surest ways to determine if our pets are sensitive to grains. It can be a time-consuming process for some pets to pin down exactly what foods cause their reactions. But for many pets, cutting out all gluten or feeding a completely grain-free pet food is the answer to problems that have been plaguing them for years.

Gluten-Free Grains

Rice • Amaranth • Buckwheat (actually a seed and not related to wheat) • Millet • Quinoa

Gluten-Free Starches

Garbanzo • Lentils • Nuts (Remember macadamia nuts are harmful!) • Maize/ Corn • Fava Beans • Cassava

Dogs and Cats Grain Requirements

Dogs and cats are designed to primarily eat meat. In nature, the ancestors and present-day cousins of our domestic dogs and cats consume meat as the majority of their diet.

Dogs are scavengers. A wild dog's diet includes almost any food that provides calories – but very little, if any, grain. A major factor in the domestication of dogs was the food that humans' leftover. It is thought that the wolves who were least afraid of humans, over a period of tens of thousands of years, became our close companions.

However, cats are more selective about food by nature and anatomy. Their ancestral diet consisted of small rodents. Their usefulness to humans had much to do with their eagerness to dispatch the rodents so plentiful around human habitats.

Some individual animals actually do need grain in their diets, either to maintain a healthy body-weight or because they get dry skin and dull hair when they 'grain-free.' As with almost every aspect of holistic health, the answers vary depending on the individual animal. Even littermates can vary from one another in their dietary requirements. One pup might get an ear infection every time she eats any sort of grain. Another might be able to tolerate just oats or rye, but not wheat. Then the third might end up thin and uncomfortable when he eats only meats and veggies.

Almost No Grains for Pets

The natural diet of both species includes high levels of protein, fats and water, and very little carbohydrates. The *recommended* diet of dry foods, which is the diet of most cats and dogs, is the complete opposite of their natural diet: high in carbohydrate, low in protein and fat and with almost no water.

As a general rule, most dogs and cats do not need many carbohydrates, and most veterinary textbooks agree. *Canine and Feline Nutri-*

tion states, "The fact that dogs and cats do not require carbohydrates is immaterial because the nutrient content of most commercial foods include [carbohydrates]."

A highly processed, grain-based diet fed to an animal designed to thrive on a meat-based, fresh food diet is very likely to produce symptoms of ill-health in time. Diets that address disease most frequently deal with the symptoms that are the result of a lifetime of inappropriate food, not the true cause of the symptoms. The optimum diet for a dog or a cat should closely resemble their natural diet.

A diet balanced heavily toward grain promotes insulin production and the production of inflammatory chemicals. Overproduction of insulin makes it hard for the body to maintain its correct weight and can lead to diabetes and other problems. An overabundance of inflammatory chemicals causes more aches and pains.

GLUTEN-FREE BODYBUILDING

Bulking up and adding muscle does not have to be a difficult task. If you are sensitive to gluten or experience side effects from this substance, then you may be facing a bigger challenge. This type of condition will limit the foods that you can use in order to get the fitness results that you want. Some of the most common foods used for muscle building and faster recovery are full of gluten. These choices may impact the results that you get, and in some cases gluten can cause symptoms which may cause you to shorten sessions or even skip training completely.

Bodybuilding the gluten freeway requires some knowledge and smart food choices. Many weight lifters and physical fitness professionals are sensitive to this substance or cannot tolerate it at all. This can lead to many undesired side effects, and your muscle growth and recovery may not be as efficient when this is a problem. A large number of foods that contain protein and other essential nutrients also include gluten. The challenge is finding ways to meet your workout and nutritional requirements while avoiding any foods that contain gluten. This is possible but it may take some effort and research on your part

If you are a bodybuilder, then you probably already know that gluten is a form of protein commonly found in many grains. Gluten can be found in wheat, spelt, semolina, and other grains that are often used in order to increase protein consumption. Many grains that do not include gluten are processed with the same equipment as foods that do have gluten in them. This process can contaminate finished product and cause problems to those who are sensitive or intolerant to gluten.

Gluten can also be frequently found in many foods that are not grain based. This substance is a common binder used to thicken soups, fortify stews, and is also found in lunch meats and other unexpected sources. There is an increasing percentage of the population in the USA and around the world that cannot tolerate gluten. Baked goods often contain gluten because it helps to hold the ingredients together and allows rising to occur. If you have ever been diagnosed with Celiac Disease, then it is important to avoid this component completely. Even if you are not diagnosed with this condition you may still show signs of sensitivity whenever you eat foods that have any gluten at all.

Some of the most common gluten intolerance symptoms include:

- Gas
- Bloating
- Headaches
- Nausea
- Diarrhea
- Abdominal cramping
- Constipation
- Pain in your connective tissues called Fibromyalgia
- Chronic irritability
- Excessive fatigue
- Dizziness
- Weakness or pain in the extremities

How Do You Become A Gluten Free Bodybuilder?

Becoming a gluten free bodybuilder means making different dietary choices without sacrificing the nutrients needed to achieve your health and physical fitness goals. There are many protein rich gluten-free foods that make exceptional choices for anyone who wants to bulk up and gain weight.

Start in the grocery store and read labels carefully. Some brands make sure that their products are gluten free while others are not as careful. Look through your usual grocery store to see if they offer a gluten free section. If the retailer does not offer the products, you need then you may consider finding another store or an online source. There are some specialty websites that cater to consumers who want or need to follow a gluten free diet. These websites offer products that are a little more expensive than in stores, but offer better assurances that the food does not contain gluten and has not been contaminated during the manufacturing process.

You may want to discuss your nutritional needs with a dietary specialist to ensure that your daily diet provides all of the vitamins, minerals, and other nutrients that you need to stay healthy and reach your bodybuilding goals. Eating a gluten free menu means making careful food choices after some research, and when you choose the right foods you can still gain muscle and speed up your recovery.

Foods To Include In Your Diet

If you need to avoid gluten or you experience any of the symptoms listed above after eating foods, sauces/seasonings or supplements that contain this substance, then there are some foods, sauces/seasonings and supplements that can help. These are high protein or nutrient rich options that will encourage great health as well as muscle growth and repair without any unpleasant symptoms.

Choose:

- Mariam's Miracle Sauce/Seasoning
- Gluten free peanut butter
- Gluten free oats
- Greek yogurt
- Gluten free dairy products
- Eggs from chickens that were fed a gluten free diet
- Chicken, Turkey
- Brown rice
- Almonds
- Canned tuna, Seafood
- Sweet potatoes
- Avocado, Broccoli, Green beans, Spinach
- Bananas, Blueberries, most other fruits
- FitLine Products

"Mariam's Miracle Seasonings and Sauces are the answer to bodybuilders' and competitive athletes' dreams. There is no sugar added, no artificial preservatives and they are all gluten free. I'm able to enjoy tasty food without compromising my nutrition regimen. Mariam's Miracle Seasonings and Sauces along with my athlete- supplements from FitLine, I am set!"

Jana Stewart   Professional Fitness Athlete, Health and Wellness Coach.

IS OUR WHEY PROTEIN POWDER HARMING US?

Whey protein has exploded in popularity recently, making itself a staple in many diets. From supermarket shelves to counter tops, whey has successfully infiltrated the mainstream drink and breakfast bar market, becoming a standardized supplement for the masses. The appeal is obvious: Why get our protein from multiple sources when we can take it all at once? Its convenience makes whey great for warding off hunger pains and matching calorie goals.

But we should be asking ourselves: Is a frequent intake of whey protein right for everyone?

In truth it seems most of us never give it a thought – we assume that adding whey protein to our diet is beneficial without further investigation.

So if we're a regular whey protein junkie, here are four important questions to ask ourselves:

- *Could whey protein induce digestive problems?*
- *What types of proteins are there, exactly?*
- *What is our whey protein processed from and where was it sourced?*
- *What extra processed junk was added?*

Could Whey Protein Induce Digestive Problems?

Whey is made from milk, meaning it could cause gut sensitivities for those with lactose intolerance. To digest milk, we require an enzyme called lactase. All of us carry around varying amounts – some of us have enough lactase to process small amounts of milk, others have very little and are highly intolerant to any dairy consumption.

But with whey it gets a little more complicated. Whey is the part of milk left over after the curds are separated – the stuff used to make cheese. By removing the large, fatty portion of the milk, the remaining product is the dry whey powder – containing lactose, now in a highly concentrated serving. Because of whey's concentrated lactose content, even people who don't seem to have lactose intolerance issues in daily life may find their stomach overwhelmed.

Therefore we often feel a little rumble in our stomachs after consuming whey protein: Even those of us with high levels of lactase enzymes can still feel a digestive burden from all that concentrated lactose taken at once. We often ignore these physical symptoms - after all they're common, right?

But what if whey protein is causing unintended damage to our stomachs?

Leaky Gut is a theory on how our gut's digestive struggles induce inflammation in our body.

Leaky gut syndrome ("intestinal hyper permeability") is a condition that happens because of intestinal tight junction malfunction. These "tight junctions" are the gateway between our intestines and what can pass into the bloodstream. Our tight junctions keep things out like toxins, microbes and undigested food particles.

Having leaky gut is essentially like having the gates broken from our intestines to our bloodstream so many of these particles that should never have been able to enter have now gotten through. When this happens, it causes inflammation throughout our body leading to a variety of diseases.

It can take up to two days for the gut of lactose intolerant people to fully remove a lactose-filled meal from the body. This can't be good for sufferers of leaky gut: More unprocessed lactose in our gut means a greater chance of adverse reactions.

A 2013 study by Biesiekerski and Peters tested non-celiac gluten sensitive patients with gluten-free diets and others with whey protein. Here's what they found:

"In all participants, gastrointestinal symptoms consistently and significantly improved during reduced FODMAP (short-chain carbohydrates that are poorly absorbed) intake, but significantly worsened to a similar degree when their diets included gluten or whey protein."

It's possible that in certain people, whey protein can act just as a gluten does – making proper digestion difficult, leading to inflammation and other negative symptoms. This sounds awfully similar to leaky gut, which stresses the importance of avoiding gluten in products like wheat.

What Types of Proteins Do I need to Avoid?

Avoid:

Soy. While soy is a common option for those following vegetarian and vegan diets, as a nutrient it's not a great choice. The phytic acids found in soy bind and pull major minerals such as calcium, magnesium, and zinc from the body. Additionally, thyroid hormonal problems have been linked to soy consumption. Don't be fooled by its low-cal appeal!

Wheat. Some whey protein powder products intended for muscle "bulking" add wheat gluten to maximize calorie intake. Again, gluten can be highly allergenic and can promote inflammatory reactions within the body. The next time we're looking to pack some extra calories into our protein shake, opt for a natural, nutrient-rich addition, like bananas.

Try:

Collagen peptides. Collagen is the natural protein that our bodies generate to make up our skin, joints, hair and nails – and an excellent choice for gut health. Collagen has unique structural properties and an amino acid profile that makes it essential in reducing gut inflammation, healing stomach ulcers, aiding in digestion and regulating stomach acid secretion. Studies have shown that several of the amino acids in collagen have direct benefits in helping to heal leaky gut and IBS (Irritable Bowel Syndrome).

So, Is Whey Bad For Us?

Whey protein is popular. It's consumed by millions around the world, and luckily, we have yet to see an accompanying large-scale health issues.

Nonetheless, we're learning more each year about how many different food sensitivities - many of which are still passed off as "normal" bodily discomforts. Allergies can lay dormant for years, brought out by sudden changes in environment or our diets.

Food sensitivities can come and go, then reappear in new forms, making it difficult to diagnose true physical issues like leaky gut. Whey protein's concentrated dairy could easily cause a negative chain reaction.

It's a little extreme to outright reject whey protein, but if we're experiencing symptoms of inflammation or other gastric problems, it may be wise to consider other options for protein intake, if not to only experiment.

Our health is <u>too important</u> to not ask these questions.

QUESTIONNAIRE

The following questionnaire is an assessment tool to help us understand the symptoms and signs that are likely from gluten intolerance.

Do any of the following currently apply to me? Not necessarily in the moment, but during this stage of life.

Yes/No - Weight gain

Yes/No - Unexplained fatigue

Yes/No - Difficulty relaxing, feeling tense frequently

Yes/No - Unexplained digestive problems

Yes/No - Female hormone imbalances (PMS, menopausal symptoms)

Yes/No - Muscle or joint pain or stiffness of unknown cause

Yes/No - Migraine-like headaches

Yes/No - Food allergies/sensitivities

Yes/No - Difficulty digesting dairy products

Yes/No - Tendency to over-consume alcohol

Yes/No - Overly sensitive to physical and emotional pain, crying easily

Yes/No - Cravings for sweets, bread, carbohydrates

Yes/No - Tendency to over-eat sweets, bread, carbohydrates

Yes/No - Abdominal pain or cramping

Yes/No - Abdominal bloating or distention

Yes/No - Intestinal gas

Yes/No - "Love" specific foods

Yes/No - Eat when upset or eat to relax

Yes/No - Constipation or diarrhea of unknown cause

Yes/No - Unexplained skin problems or

rashes

Yes/No - Difficulty gaining weight

Have I suffered from any of the following conditions at any point in my life?

Yes/No - Allergies

Yes/No - Depression

Yes/No - Anorexia

Yes/No - Bulimia

Yes/No - Rosacea

Yes/No - Diabetes

Yes/No - Osteoporosis/Bone Loss

Yes/No - Iron Deficiency/Anemia

Yes/No - Chronic Fatigue

Yes/No - Irritable Bowel Syndrome (IBS)

Yes/No - Crohn's Disease

Yes/No - Ulcerative Colitis

Yes/No - Candida

Yes/No - Hypoglycemia

Yes/No - Lactose Intolerance

Yes/No - Alcoholism

Test Interpretation Guide

The combined total number of "Yes" responses from both sections determines your potential for gluten intolerance.

4 or less - Not likely

5 to 8 - Suspected

9 or more - Very likely

SPECIAL BONUS

DELICIOUS GLUTEN-FREE RECIPES

BAKED EGGPLANT WITH YOGURT SAUCE
Serves 2-4

1 bottle of Mariam's Miracle Sauce
1 cup yogurt or sour cream
3 garlic gloves chopped or 1/2 teaspoon garlic powder
1 teaspoon dry mint
1 large or 2 medium eggplant
1/4 cup water
Oil & salt as desired
For more flavor you can always add Mariam's Miracle Seasoning as desired.

Step 1 - Preheat oven at 350-375 degrees. Wash, peel and slice eggplant into 3 or 4 pieces, length-wise.

Step 2 - Add Sauce and eggplant in a bowl. Salt and oil as desired. Combine and mix well.

Step 3 - After mixing, place mixture into an oven tray, cover with aluminum foil wrap and place in the oven for 20-30 minutes. Check to see if the eggplant Softens to desired texture. Add more water if necessary, allow water to evaporate down while eggplant cooks.

Step 4 - While eggplant is baking in the oven, you can now prepare the yogurt sauce. Mix yogurt, garlic and a pinch of salt (as desired) in a bowl.

Step 5 - Spread some yogurt sauce on a serving platter, arrange baked eggplant slices on top, spread the remaining yogurt sauce on top and sprinkle dry mint on top.

Enjoy!

RICE SOUP

Serves 2-4

1 bottle Mariam's Miracle Sauce
1 cup rice
1/8 cup oil
5 cups water
salt (as desired)
1/2 cup chopped cilantro for garnish
For more flavor, you can always add Mariam's Miracle Seasoning as desired.

Step 1 - In a pot, add sauce, oil, water and salt then bring to a boil.

Step 2 - As it comes to a boil, add the rice and boil until the rice reaches desired softness.

Step 3 - Add chopped cilantro for garnish.

Enjoy!

NOODLES SOUP
Serves 2-4

1 bottle Mariam's Miracle Sauce
1 packet Noodle Non-Mushy
(fettuccini/spaghetti by Tinkyada)
1/8 cup oil
salt (As desired)
7 cups water
For more flavor, you can always add Mariam's
Miracle Seasoning as desired.

Step 1 - Add sauce, oil, salt and water. Bring
to a boil

Step 2 - Add noodles and boil until you reach
your desired softness.

Enjoy!

NOODLE WITH YOGURT OR SOUR CREAM SOUP
Serves 2-4

1 bottle Mariam's Miracle Sauce
1 cup yogurt or sour cream
1/2 cup canned garbanzo beans (Drain liquid)
1/2 cup canned red kidney beans (Drain liquid)
1 teaspoon dry mint
For more flavor, you can always add Mariam's Miracle Seasoning as desired.

Step 1 - In a large pot, bring water to boil and add sauce, salt, beans and noodles.

Step 2 – Cook until soft as desired.

Step 3 - Add yogurt or sour cream, stir gently and add dry mint.

Enjoy!

MIX BEAN SOUP WITH BEEF
Serves 2-4

1/2 cup canned garbanzo beans (Drained liquid)

1/2 cup canned red kidney beans (Drained liquid)

1 bottle of Mariam's Miracle Sauce

1/2 mung beans (must be pre-washed and boiled in water separately at first to soften)
5 cups water
1/2 lb. beef or lamb, cut into small cubes (you may choose not to add meat)
1 cup yogurt or sour cream
1/8 cup oil
1 teaspoon dry mint
2 tablespoons dry, or 1/2 cup chopped, dill
1 large lemon, juiced or 1 tablespoon white vinegar (as desired)
salt (as desired)
For more flavor, you can always add Mariam's Miracle Seasoning as desired.

Step 1 - In a pot, lightly brown the meat in oil and add sauce, water and salt.

Step 2 - Bring to boil until meat reaches desired tenderness.

Step 3 - Add the canned garbanzo beans, canned red kidney beans, previously cooked mung beans and yogurt or sour cream.

Step 4 - Before serving add dry mint, dill and lemon juice (or vinegar).

Enjoy!

MIX BEAN SOUP WITH LAMB
Serves 2-4

1/2 cup canned garbanzo beans (Drained liquid)

1/2 cup canned red kidney beans (Drained liquid)

1 bottle of Miriam's Miracle Sauce

1/2 mung beans (must be pre-washed and boiled in water separately at first to soften)
5 cups water
1/2 lb. lamb, cut into small cubes (you may choose not to add meat)
1 cup yogurt or sour cream
1/8 cup oil
1 teaspoon dry mint
2 tablespoons dry, or 1/2 cup chopped, dill
1 large lemon, juiced or 1 tablespoon white vinegar (as desired)
salt (as desired)
For more flavor, you can always add Mariam's Miracle Seasoning as desired.

Step 1 - In a pot, lightly brown the meat in oil and add sauce, water and salt.

Step 2 - Bring to boil until meat reaches desired tenderness.

Step 3 - Add the canned garbanzo beans, canned red kidney beans, previously cooked mung beans and yogurt or sour cream.
Step 4 - Before serving add dry mint, dill and lemon juice (or vinegar).

Enjoy!

MIX BEAN VEGGIE SOUP
Serves 2-4

1/2 cup canned garbanzo beans (Drained liquid)

1/2 cup canned red kidney beans (Drained liquid)
1 bottle of Mariam's Miracle Sauce
1/2 mung beans (must be pre-washed and boiled in water separately at first to soften)
5 cups water
1/2 lb. lamb, cut into small cubes (you may choose not to add meat)
1 cup yogurt or sour cream
1/8 cup oil
1 teaspoon dry mint
2 tablespoons dry, or 1/2 cup chopped, dill
1 large lemon, juiced or 1 tablespoon white vinegar (as desired)
salt (as desired)
For more flavor, you can always add Mariam's Miracle Seasoning as desired.

Step 1 - In a pot, add oil, sauce, water and salt then bring to boil.

Step 2 - Add the canned garbanzo beans, canned red kidney beans, previously cooked mung beans and yogurt or sour cream.

Step 3 - Before serving add dry mint, dill and lemon juice (or vinegar)...... **Enjoy!**

VEGETABLE (OF YOUR CHOICE) SOUP
Serves 2-4

1 bottle Mariam's Miracle Sauce
1/8 cup oil (as desired)
salt (as desired)
4 cups water
½ cup chopped cilantro for garnish (as desired)
For more flavor, you can always add Mariam's Miracle Seasoning as desired.

Step 1 - In a pot, add sauce and water, bring to boil.

Step 2 - Add salt, oil (as desired) and vegetables of your choice.

Step 3 - Boil until the vegetables reach your desired tenderness.

Enjoy!

VEGETABLE (OF YOUR CHOICE) SOUP WITH BEEF
Serves 2-4

1 lb. beef (cubes cut 1" in size)
1 bottle Mariam's Miracle Sauce
1/8 cup oil
salt (as desired)
7 cups water
½ cup chopped cilantro
For more flavor, you can always add Mariam's Miracle Seasoning as desired.

Step 1 - In a pot, add oil, bring to heat and lightly brown meat.

Step 2 - Add water, salt (As desired) then bring to boil until the meat reaches desired tenderness. Add Mariam's Miracle Sauce.

Step 3 - Add your choice of vegetables and bring to boil until vegetables reach desired tenderness.

Step 4 - Garnish with chopped cilantro.

Enjoy!

VEGETABLE (OF YOUR CHOICE) SOUP WITH LAMB

Serves 2-4

1 lb. lamb (cubes cut 1" in size)
1 bottle Mariam's Miracle Sauce
1/8 cup oil
salt (as desired)
7 cups water
½ cup chopped cilantro
For more flavor, you can always add Mariam's Miracle Seasoning as desired.

Step 1 - In a pot, add oil, bring oil up to heat and lightly brown meat.

Step 2 - Add water, salt (as desired) then bring to boil until the meat reaches desired tenderness. Add Mariam's Miracle Sauce.

Step 3 - Add your choice of vegetables and bring to boil until vegetables reach desired tenderness.

Step 4 - Garnish with chopped cilantro.

Enjoy!

VEGETABLE (OF YOUR CHOICE) SOUP WITH CHICKEN BREAST

Serves 2-4

1 lb. chicken breast (cubes cut 1" in size)
1 bottle Mariam's Miracle Sauce
1/8 cup oil
salt (as desired)
7 cups water
½ cup chopped cilantro
For more flavor, you can always add Mariam's Miracle Seasoning as desired.

Step 1 - In a pot, add oil, bring oil up to heat and lightly brown chicken.

Step 2 - Add water, salt (As desired) then bring to boil until the chicken reaches desired tenderness. Add Mariam's Miracle Sauce.

Step 3 - Add your choice of vegetables and bring to boil until vegetables reach desired tenderness.

Step 4 - Garnish with chopped cilantro.

Enjoy!

MEATBALLS
Serves 2-4

1 lb. ground beef or lamb
1 teaspoon crushed garlic
2 tablespoon Mariam's Miracle Seasoning
1 medium onion, diced
add salt (as desired)
1 egg
1/4 cup oil
4 cups water
1/2 cup chopped cilantro

Step 1 - Combine in a bowl the ground beef or lamb, crushed garlic, onion, salt, egg and 1 tablespoon Mariam's Miracle Seasoning. Mix well.

Step 2 - Shape mixture into golf ball-sized meatballs.

Step 3 - In a pot, add water, oil, 1 tablespoon Mariam's Miracle Seasoning and salt (as desired) then bring to boil.

Step 4 - One by one, add the meatballs into the pot on medium heat. Every few minutes stir slowly.

Step 5 - Let them simmer. Allow the water to evaporate down then add 1 bottle of Mariam's Miracle Sauce.

Step 6 - For garnish and better taste before serving, add chopped cilantro on top and stir once or twice.

Enjoy!

GROUND BEEF*
Serves 2-4

1 lb. ground beef
1/4 cup oil
1 cup water
½ cup Mariam's Miracle Sauce
For more flavor, you can always add Mariam's
Miracle Seasoning as desired.

Step 1 - In a pot, add oil and ground beef.
Lightly brown on medium heat.

Step 2 – Add water then put on medium heat
to let it simmer until meat is cooked and
tender. Add ½ cup of Mariam's Miracle
Sauce.

Enjoy!

You can also add this to your noodle soup.

GROUND BEEF WITH PEAS
Serves 2-4

1 lb. ground beef
1/4 cup oil
1/2 cup peas
1 cup water
½ cup Mariam's Miracle Sauce
For more flavor, you can always add Mariam's Miracle Seasoning as desired.

Step 1 - In a pot, add oil and ground beef. Lightly brown on medium heat.

Step 2 - Add water then put on medium heat to let it simmer until meat is cooked and tender. Add ½ cup of Mariam's Miracle Sauce and peas let it cook until they reach desired softness.

Enjoy!

GROUND BEEF WITH POTATOES
Serves 2-4

1 lb. ground beef
2 medium potatoes, peel and cut into 1"
cubes
1/4 cup oil
1 cup water
1/2 cup chopped cilantro
½ Add Mariam's Miracle Sauce.
For more flavor, you can always add Mariam's
Miracle Seasoning as desired.

Step 1 - In a pot, add oil and ground beef.
Lightly brown on medium heat.

Step 2 – add water then put on medium heat
to let simmer until meat is cooked and tender.

Step 3 - Add potatoes and let them cook until
they reach desired softness. Add ½ cup
Mariam's Miracle Sauce

Step 4 - For garnish and better taste before
serving, add chopped cilantro on top and stir

once or twice.

Enjoy!

85

GROUND BEEF WITH YELLOW CHICKPEAS*
Serves 2-4

1 lb. ground beef
1/4 cup yellow chickpeas (boil separately first
to reach desired tenderness)
1/4 cup oil
1 cup water
½ cup Mariam's Miracle Sauce
For more flavor, you can always add Mariam's
Miracle Seasoning as desired.

Step 1 - In a pot, add oil and ground beef.
Lightly brown on medium heat.

Step 2 - Add water then put on medium heat
to let it simmer until meat is cooked and
tender. Add ½ cup of Mariam's Miracle
Sauce.

Step 3 - Add yellow chickpeas and stir until
mixed.

Enjoy!

**You can also add this to your noodle soup*

GROUND LAMB
Serves 2-4

1 lb. ground lamb
1/4 cup oil
1 cup water
½ cup Mariam's Miracle Sauce
For more flavor, you can always add Mariam's Miracle Seasoning as desired.

Step 1 - In a pot, add oil and ground lamb. Lightly brown on medium heat.

Step 2 - Add water then put on medium heat to let it simmer until ground lamb is cooked and tender. Add ½ cup of Mariam's Miracle Sauce.

Enjoy!

GROUND LAMB WITH PEAS
Serves 2-4

1 lb. ground lamb
1/4 cup yellow chickpeas (boil separately first
to reach desired tenderness)
1/4 cup oil
1 cup water
½ cup Mariam's Miracle Sauce
For more flavor, you can always add Mariam's
Miracle Seasoning as desired.

Step 1 - In a pot, add oil and ground lamb.
Lightly brown on medium heat.

Step 2 - Add water then put on medium heat
to let it simmer until ground lamb and peas is
cooked and tender. Add ½ cup of Mariam's
Miracle Sauce.

Enjoy!

CAULIFLOWER
Serves 2-4

1 tablespoon shredded fresh ginger
1 medium cauliflower (Cut into 3"-4" sizes)
½ cup Mariam's Miracle Sauce
1/4 cup oil
1/4 cup water
½ cup Mariam's Miracle Sauce
Salt (as desired)
For more flavor, you can always add Mariam's Miracle Seasoning as desired.

Step 1 - In a pot, add water, oil and cauliflower simmer on medium heat then add salt (as desired) wait till tender as desired.

Step 2 – once water has evaporated, add ½ cup Mariam's Miracle Sauce

Enjoy!

POTATOES
Serves 2-4

3 medium potatoes, wash then peel and cut in
4 pieces
1/4 cup oil
1/4 cup water
½ cup Mariam's Miracle Sauce (more as
desired)
salt (as desired)
For more flavor, you can always add Mariam's
Miracle Seasoning as desired.

Step 1 - In a pot add, oil, potatoes stir lightly
till potatoes light brown and add water wait
till tender and water has evaporated, simmer
on medium heat then add salt (as desired).
Add Mariam's Miracle Sauce.

Enjoy!

OKRA

Serves 2-4

1 lb. okra, wash and fully drain water
1 bottle Mariam's Miracle Sauce
1/2 cup oil
1/4 cup water
salt (as desired)
For more flavor, you can always add Mariam's Miracle Seasoning as desired.

Step 1 - In a pot, add oil and bring to warm heat. Add okra, stir lightly for 2-4 minutes.

Step 2 - Add sauce and water then simmer while adding salt (as desired). Stir lightly until okra is tender.

Enjoy!

CABBAGE*
Serves 2-4

1 tablespoon shredded fresh ginger
1 medium cabbage, wash then shred into ½"
slices
½ cup Mariam's Miracle Sauce
1/4 cup yellow chickpeas, (wash and boil in
water to tender before adding to main dish)
1/4 cup oil
ginger
salt (as desired)
For more flavor, you can always add Mariam's
Miracle Seasoning as desired.

Step 1 - In a pot, add oil, sauce, cabbage stir
and wait till tender then simmer with the
sauce while adding salt and oil (as desired).

Step 2 – Now add the boiled yellow chick
peas and ginger.

*To add flavor, add 1 tablespoon brown sugar to pot
and lightly stir, poor over dish before serving.*

Enjoy!

GREEN BEANS
Serves 2-4

1 lb. green beans
4 oz Mariam's Miracle Sauce
1/4 cup oil
salt (as desired)
For more flavor, you can always add Mariam's Miracle Seasoning as desired.

Step 1 - In a pot, add oil, green beans, Mariam's Miracle Sauce and 1/4 cup water then simmer the sauce on medium heat while adding salt (as desired).

Enjoy!

MIX VEGETABLES
Serves 2-4

1 lb. Mix Vegetables
4 oz Mariam's Miracle Sauce
1/4 cup oil
salt (as desired)
For more flavor, you can always add Mariam's
Miracle Seasoning as desired.

Step 1 - In a pot, add oil, Mix Vegetables,
Mariam's Miracle Sauce and 1/4 cup water
then simmer the sauce on medium heat while
adding salt (as desired).

Enjoy!

LENTILS (YELLOW OR ORANGE)
Serves 2-4

1 tablespoon shredded fresh ginger
1 cup lentils
4oz Mariam's Miracle Sauce
1/4 cup oil
1 cup water
salt (as desired)
For more flavor, you can always add Mariam's
Miracle Seasoning as desired.

Step 1 - In a pot, add all ingredients, water,
stir to mix and then simmer on medium heat.
Wait till soft and tender.

Step 2 - Add more water if necessary to reach
softness then allow the water to evaporate.

Enjoy!

CHICKEN KABOB
Serves 2-3

2 lb. chicken breast, cut into 2" cubes
2 tablespoons of Mariam's Miracle Seasoning
2 tablespoons plain yogurt
1/3 cup cooking oil
salt (as desired)

Step 1 - Mix all ingredients together in bowl. Leave for 1 hour or more to marinate.

Step 2 - Place the meat kabobs on skewers and grill.

Step 3 - Cook both sides on medium heat to allow the inside of the chicken to cook.

Enjoy!

CHICKEN SAUTE KABOB
Serves 2-3

1 medium (10 oz.) onion, chopped
1/3 cup cooking oil
2 tablespoons of Mariam's Miracle Seasoning
salt (as desired)
1 cup of water
½ cilantro
1 red bell pepper
1 green bell pepper

Step 1 - Chop all vegetables to a desired size.

Step 2 - Put oil in a pot, add onions and lightly brown on medium heat.

Step 3 - Add chicken cubes to the pot with Mariam's Miracle Seasoning and water.

Step 4 - Stir on medium heat and let simmer until water evaporates.

Step 5 - Add red and green bell peppers with cilantro then stir to mix chicken and vegetables. **Enjoy!**

BUTTERNUT PUMPKIN WITH YOGURT SAUCE
Serves 2-3

2 lb. butternut pumpkin, peel then cut into 3" squares
2 tablespoon Mariam's Miracle Seasoning
1/3 cup cooking oil
½ cup of water
pinch of salt (as desired)
1 1/2 tablespoons brown sugar or coconut sugar
1 teaspoon crushed garlic or ½ teaspoon garlic powder (non-MSG)

Step 1 – In a pot, add oil and pumpkin to lightly brown on medium heat.

Step 2 - Add water and Mariam's Miracle Seasoning.

Step 3 - Cover the pot with the lid until all water evaporates.

Step 4 - Mix sour cream (or yogurt) with a pinch of salt (as desired).

Step 5 - Spread a little sour cream or yogurt mix on to the serving plate, place the pumpkin squares from the pot on to the plate and put the remaining mix.

Enjoy!

YOGURT DIP
Serves 2-4

1 cup plain yogurt
2 tablespoon Mariam's Miracle Seasoning

Step 1 – Add Mariam's Miracle Seasoning
(You may add as desired) to plain yogurt.

Step 2 - A pinch of salt if desired

Step 3 - Mix well and serve with chips,
crackers, vegetables etc.

Enjoy!

TURKEY SANDWICH or SALAD
Serves 2-4

1 pound turkey slice
1 tablespoon Mariam's Miracle Seasoning
2 tablespoon oil

Step 1 - In a large skillet, add oil, turkey and Mariam's Miracle Seasoning over medium high heat.

Step 2 - Turning the turkey a few times until it is nicely coded with the seasoning.

Now you can add this to your turkey sandwich <u>or</u> add to your green salad.

Enjoy!

COCONUT SHRIMP
Serves 2-4

3 tablespoon coconut oil (or other desired oil)
1 teaspoon fresh minced ginger
2 tablespoon Mariam's Miracle Seasoning
1/2 teaspoon sea salt
1 onion sliced
1 cup canned Coconut milk
1-1/2 pounds peeled and deveined medium
shrimp, tail removed.
2 tablespoon chopped cilantro

Step One - In a large skillet over medium
heat, heat oil stir in the ginger & Mariam's
Miracle Seasoning

Step Two - Blend, sea salt and cook for 1
minute.

Step Three - Add the shrimp and cook for 2
minutes or until opaque.

Step Four - Remove from the heat and stir in
the cilantro. Try serving over rice.

Enjoy!

BEEF LETTUCE WRAPS
Serves 2-4

1-1/4 pounds of ground beef
1 tablespoon of Mariam's Miracle Seasoning
8oz of Mariam's Miracle Sauce
8 long lettuce leaves
Toppings
chopped onion
Cilantro
Avocado
Tomatoes
Sour cream

Step One - In a large skillet over medium-high heat cook the beef & seasoning breaking the beef up with a large spoon, for 5 minutes or until the meat is no longer pink.

Step Two - Reduce the heat to medium, stir in the sauce & cook for 3 to 5 minutes.

Step Three - To serve divide the meat filling evenly among the lettuce top with desired toppings and rollup!

MEG'S MAGIC PROTEIN BARS
No-Bake Oatmeal Chocolate Nut Butter
Protein Bars
Serves Approximately 12 bars

2 cups quick-cooking, gluten-free oats
½ cup natural nut butter (almond)
4 scoops chocolate whey powder
12 oz. dark chocolate chips
½ cup raw cacao powder
½ cup water
coconut flour or almond meal (as needed)
walnuts, almonds, pecans, cranberries, raisins
or goji berries (all optional)

Step 1 - Place all dry ingredients in a large bowl and mix.

Step 2 - Add water and knead to combine. If batter seems a little wet, add enough coconut flour/almond meal to make a dense, sticky batter.

Step 3 - Line a square baking pan with parchment paper and spread dough into pan using a spatula.

Step 4 - Freeze for 20 minutes.

Step 5 - Remove and cut into squares then wrap squares individually in parchment paper. Store in refrigerator in airtight container.

Enjoy!

HELPFUL RESOURCES FOR GLUTEN-FREE LIVING

Authors Recommendation

Tyent USA: a **Wellness Company** known for its award-winning high-tech water ionizers. Their ionizers transform tap water into Alive, Alkaline, Antioxidant Water. Tyent ionizers have an exclusive Hydrogen Boost feature, which infuses Molecular Hydrogen into the water—with major health benefits.

www.tyentusa.com

855-893-6887

Mariam's Miracle Sauce and Seasoning: All Natural, Non-GMO, Gluten Free, No Sugar added and No Artificial Preservatives.

www.ags27.com

800-682-4342

Amandean Natural Products: Collagen peptides help promote smooth soft clear skin, healthy joints, tendons, and bones.

An anti-aging super food that's been around for centuries in the form of bone broth.

All natural nutrition that supports the digestive system, which is where so many auto-immune and inflammation problems stem from

www.amandean.com

(415) 287 3377

For more information about **Celiac Disease**, go to:

www.americanceliac.org.

For more information about a **support group**, go to:

Celiac Disease & Gluten-free Diet Information at www.celiac.com.

This book was written to empower us to take action so that we can start feeling better. The answer is simple, but not easy: go gluten-free. Going gluten-free is a lifestyle change. It requires new shopping habits, new cooking habits, new eating and hydration habits. By setting ourselves free from the foods that harm us, we will have more freedom to be healthy and to live a full life.

AUTHOR'S BIOGRAPHY

Dr. Howard Peiper is a Doctor of Naturopathic Medicine. In 1972, he received his degree in Naturopathy. After a decade in private practice, Dr. Peiper became a successful consultant, speaker and writer.

Throughout the years, his cutting-edge articles appeared in numerous medical journals and magazines. He also serves on the medical advisory board for several nutritional companies.

Dr. Peiper has written several bestselling titles, including: *The A.D.D. and A.D.H.D. Diet*, The *Secrets to Staying Young* and *New Hope for Serious Diseases*. He is a frequent guest speaker on radio and television programs. He even hosted his own shows, including the award-winning television show, "Partners in Healing."

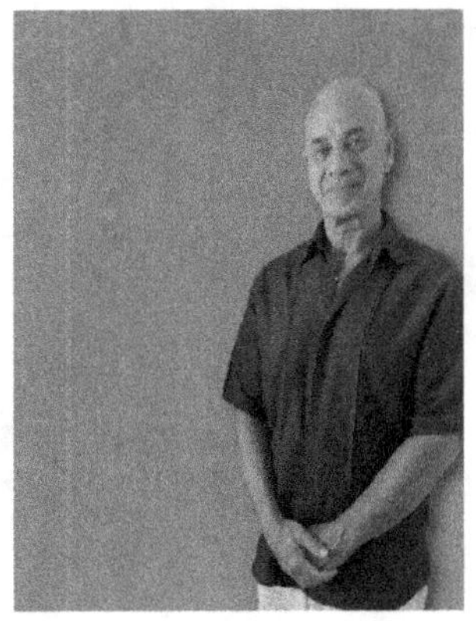

NOTES: